# Alkaline Diet

Ultimate Guide for Beginners - Naturally Lose Weight, Reverse Disease and Gain Unlimited Energy

including, but not limited to, — errors, omissions, or inaccuracies.

# Table of Contents

# Introduction

Over the past years, there have been a number of different diet plans introduced into the market. Some of these diet plans have managed to make a big impact while others faded within a few months of gaining popularity.

When it comes to weight loss, people often look for the more convenient methods to get fit rather than something that can benefit the body. If you want to lose weight, then your main motto shouldn't just be to burn fat but also to get healthy and prevent the risk of a number of diseases from occurring. You have to follow a healthy diet plan that works well on your body and mind, and also helps you stay healthy by lowering the risk of some of the most chronic illnesses which people suffer from when they do not pay attention to their health.

The reason an alkaline diet has gained so much popularity is because it focuses not only on weight loss but on decreasing the risk of diseases that are caused due to lack of nutrients and antioxidants in the body. The diet plan that Dr. Sebi introduced not only managed to prove effective when applied to your daily lifestyle, but it also turned out to be an easy diet plan to follow as soon as your body got used to it.

This detailed guide gives you hands-on information about an alkaline diet, what you need in order to follow the diet, and how it can benefit you with a few changes in your lifestyle. You will also understand why Dr. Sebi encourages people to adapt to veganism. This guide will help you transform your mind body and soul!

# Chapter 1 - What Is Alkalinity? Why Should I Care?

It's no hidden secret that certain foods work well on your body while others have bad side effects. But the key to understanding which food is healthy for you and what kind of food you need to avoid is important because in between a burger and a salad, there is a lot of room for you to introduce healthier options that can help your body heal from within and make you look great at the same time.

The one factor that helps you to understand how healthy you are is figuring out whether you have an alkaline body or an acidic body. If you have a high acidic level, then you need to understand how you can alkalize your body to lead a healthy lifestyle.

When you suffer from high acidic levels in your body, you are more prone to problems such as fatigue or low energy levels. Other signs of high acid levels in your body also include brittle nails and hair. It is also known to cause low bone density and osteoporosis in women which can cause multiple fractures with a simple fall. Although people do not take acidic levels in their body that seriously - and they should, it also results in heavy breathing and weight gain, which is often followed by obesity. An acidic diet can also introduce digestive issues along with diabetes. People with high acidic levels are also known to suffer from skin related problems and acne, and have a low immune system which means they are more susceptible to infections and allergies. These people are also at a higher risk of heart problems and cancer. If you want to stay away from these problems, it's important for you to transform your body into an alkaline body by following a healthy diet.

## What Is Alkalinity?

An alkaline diet is based on the content of alkalinity in your body. Your alkalinity levels are measured by figuring out whether you have higher alkaline content or higher acidic content in your body. While the total alkalinity in your body means having a high pH level, the truth is while pH levels are a part of an alkaline diet, it does not make up the diet completely. For instance, alkalinity in a body is measured by the amount of Alkaline substances present in the water content in your body. The normal pH level for alkalinity is anything between 0 to 14. If you have a pH level that is higher than 7, your body is neutral and if it's lower than 7, this means you have more acidic content in your system.

Anything above 7 indicates higher alkalinity levels while below 7 indicates acidic levels in the body. It is important for every person to understand the level of alkalinity in the body because a diet plan is to be based on the pH level of the individual. If your pH levels are very low, you need to make sure you stay away from acidic food and also make sure that you consume nutritious foods. Most people today have high acidic content in the system which is why focusing on an alkaline diet is something you need to consider doing. Foods such as meat and fresh dairy, eggs, grain, and alcohol all contain high acidic levels that aren't great for the body. Neutral foods are usually natural fats, sugar and starches which also need to be avoided. An alkaline diet is basically a diet that is filled with fruits, legumes, and vegetables. These are the kind of foods you need to focus on eating to get healthy.

## What Exactly Does "pH Level" Mean?

The term pH is not new and you have probably heard it numerous times in your classroom during a science class. The pH scale is basically used to measure the alkalinity or acidity in any substance where 7 is considered to be the neutral number and anything above it is alkaline where is anything below it is acidic. To measure the alkalinity or acidity in a substance, you need an aqueous solution. Human blood is aqueous because it contains high water content and this means that there is a pH level in your blood as well. This doesn't mean you can test the pH level in your blood because the pH level in your blood will not change except for when you are in a critical situation and have a life-threatening disease.

The alkaline levels in your saliva and urine however keep changing depending on the kind of food that you eat, and this enables you to understand your cellular health. The reason this is important is because without monitoring the cellular level, you will not manage to figure out whether you are healthy or not.

While the pH levels in your blood usually clock under 7, the levels in urine could go as low as 3. To begin following a healthy alkaline diet, you need to understand how long your levels of alkalinity are. This will help you figure out what needs to be changed and how you have to make the changes.

The reason monitoring your pH levels is important is because when it goes considerably low, your body turns acidic and you could even suffer from something known as chronic low-grade acidosis. This is normally caused when there is a high consumption of acidic foods that impact your body and results in low calcium, potassium, magnesium, and mineral levels in your body.

Research has proven that following an alkaline diet can help reduce multiple health-related problems and aid in effective weight loss. This is why it's important for you to understand how the pH levels in your body impact your overall health.

## What Is The Alkaline Diet?

An alkaline diet is a diet that helps lower the acidic levels in your body by maintaining the pH balance. Therefore you lose weight and get healthier, lowering the risk of multiple diseases. This diet had gained a lot of popularity when Dr. Sebi openly spoke about how effective it is and how incorporating the diet plan into your daily routine can help you lead a longer and more fruitful life.

Figuring out an alkaline diet could cause a lot of confusion because this diet may seem very complicated when you take a glance. In theory, an alkaline diet is a diet that helps lower your body's acidic levels. This may seem like a bit tough to understand but when you start consuming fruits that have higher alkaline content and lower acidic content, it is obvious that your body starts healing. This will make it come closer to a healthy alkaline level rather than an acidic one. There are tons of food that reduce a lot of acid in your body and people are so used to consuming these foods on a regular basis, they don't realize what's affecting their body. Following a regular diet plan may seem like the perfect solution because it reflects on your weighing scale and you even notice that you have lost a few pounds. However, that doesn't necessarily mean you are getting any healthier. If you want to stay healthy, you have to lower the risk of diseases in your system and keep your vital organs functioning effectively. That's what an alkaline diet does to you which is why once people understand how effective the diet plan is, they start adapting towards leading an alkaline lifestyle and avoiding foods that have high acidic content.

## Testing Yourself For Acidity

Once you have decided you want to follow the alkaline diet, you need to start planning the small changes in your lifestyle one step at a time. Taking a plunge into the first diet plan you see is not the ideal solution because everybody is different and for you to make the most out of this diet plan, you need to understand your pH level before you move forward. To do this, you need to test your acid levels and see just how high the acidic level is.

Testing for acidic levels in your body is very simple. You need to get a pH test paper. This paper tests the acid and alkaline levels of any liquid and you can either use urine or saliva to test your acidic levels. However, it is highly recommended that you test it with the first urine you collect in the morning after at least 6 hours of uninterrupted sleep. To do the test, all you need to do is take a strip of the paper and dip it into a cup of urine you have accumulated or urinate directly on the paper. If you are not comfortable urinating, you can then spit on the paper as soon as you get up in the morning.

When you purchase the pH paper, it comes with a color chart to help you figure out just how acidic or basic your body is. The colors usually range from yellow to blue and they have numbers written by their side. As mentioned earlier, if you are below seven, it means you are on the acidic side but if you are above 7, you are healthy.

There is more sense to purchase the pH test paper and use it every now and then. The reason being once you incorporate the diet plan you will manage to measure results on a regular basis and this helps keep your motivation levels high.

**Signs Your Body Is Too Acidic**

While it may be easy to get pH testing paper from various shopping websites all over the internet, in case you haven't managed to find this test strip yet, you can always look out for the early warning signs. These signs will tell if your body is too acidic and you need to take charge for you to live a healthy life.

1. One of the major signs that your body is too acidic is when you start feeling too tired even if you've rested for over 8

hours every night. People who have a high acid content in their system tend to feel tired and low on energy even with enough rest.

2. High acidic levels in your body also make you feel sad and depressed most of the time. Even it is a reason to celebrate and you still can't feel genuinely happy, this could be a sign that you have high acidic levels in your body.

3. People who suffer from high acidic levels also tend to get irritable for no apparent reason and they snap very easily. If you are told that you are snappy or irritable, this could be because you have high acidic levels.

4. Another common sign that you have high acidic levels is the inability to focus effectively on your task. If you find it difficult to get your mind in one place

and get a job done effectively, this is another sign that your acidic levels are high and it needs to be brought down under control.

5. Low immunity levels and the susceptibility to infections such as cold and flu is another common sign of a high acidic level.

6. People who also suffer from skin problems and dry skin, even during warmer months of the year, could have a high acidic level.

7. Hormonal imbalance is another sign that you need to be on the lookout for.

8. Another common problem involves digestive issues which could be a combination of constipation along with diarrhea.

9. Shortness of breath, chronic pain, sensitivity in teeth and gums and a stiff

neck are also common signs that your body is too acidic and you need to do something to change it.

These are some of the early signs and the sooner you identify them, the better it is because you will manage to shift towards a healthy diet plan.

# Chapter 2 - Who Was Dr. Sebi?

Dr. Sebi happens to be the inspiration behind the alkaline diet. He was known to be a herbalist and intracellular therapist and a natural healer who was native to Honduras. His diet is inspired by his native land and includes a ton of alkaline foods which are natural and help curb the side effects of high acidic levels in the body.

He designed the diet plan after extensive research and understanding how much trouble acidic levels caused to the body, and why it's necessary to protect the body against acid levels and mucus, that later develop into various diseases. His teachings have managed to enrich the lives of many and helped them to promote healthy living. The alkaline diet plan he came up with not only paved the path toward healing the most life-threatening diseases, but also helped to control the risk related to those diseases. It also helped people to cope with the disease more effectively. The alkaline diet not only works well for weight loss but it has also proven to be beneficial in curing diseases such as diabetes, epilepsy, lupus, cancer, and even HIV.

The main focus of Dr. Sebi's diet was to reduce the amount of acidic foods you consume because this helps to make it difficult for diseases to thrive in your body. Dr. Sebi invested over 40 years researching how alkaline foods can promote healthy living and he finally came up with a diet plan that works well not only to lose weight but to heal your system from within.

# History

Dr. Sebi led a controversial life, and a number of people believed his teachings were not beneficial in any way. He was bold enough to come out in the open and say that he can find the cure to deadly diseases like cancer, AIDS, and diabetes that hadn't been found after all the years of medical research. His main motto was to convince people to lead a healthy life and understand the importance of alkaline foods in the regular diet.

Dr. Sebi received a lot of backlash and people believed he was trying to dupe them and force them to lead a vegan life. But once he made people understand just how effective his methods were, not only did he gain celebrity following but he also became one of the most popular herbalists you could find.

Amongst the various accusations Dr. Sebi had against him, there was one that went up to the Supreme Court. This accusation was against an advertisement he released in 1988 for claiming to cure people of deadly diseases. The court believed they had a strong case and they wanted to put him away. However, a staggering 77 people came into the court saying that they were cured after following Dr. Sebi's advice and incorporating his food into their lifestyle. As per the witnesses, 77 people declared he was not guilty and they also proved that his diet plan turned out to be a medical miracle and he was underrated.

Life moved on and people never forgot about Dr. Sebi and what an amazing healer he was. All his life he tried to make as many people understand the importance of an alkaline diet so that they could keep their diseases away.

## Philosophy On Eating Natural Foods

According to Dr. Sebi, there is a wide variety of plant-based food that you should focus on eating. Although he believes veganism is a smart way to get rid of all your health problems, he does not force you to follow such a diet. The core focus of this alkaline diet is that you eat natural and healthy foods, which enables your body to lower the acidic level and helps you heal from within.

The main philosophy of adopting an alkaline diet is so that your metabolic system starts functioning effectively once again. When your body has high contents of acid inside of it, it affects the metabolic system and this means that your body uses most of the food that you eat to be stored as fat rather than convert it into energy. When your acid levels are right at the top, it is difficult for your metabolism to work effectively and this causes a problem with the overall digestive system. If you want to start living a healthy life, you have to begin eating food that works to enhance digestion for your bodily functions to work systematically. The first stage is for your metabolism to start increasing and to convert the food you eat into energy rather than storing it in your body as fat.

When you start eating healthy foods, your pH level starts balancing out. This process takes time but it slowly and surely gets you leaning towards an alkaline way of life which benefits you in the long run. The philosophy of natural food is to ensure that you do not skip meals to lose weight but rather to include foods that are high in calcium and magnesium as well as natural fat in order to alkalize your body. There are a number of benefits you get when you follow a healthy natural diet and this not only reflects in your appearance but you also start feeling a lot better.

## Veganism

It's no secret that alkaline diet promotes veganism and encourages people to go vegan so that they can stay healthy. Although it is recommended to become a vegan while you follow the alkaline diet, it's not compulsory and if your body can handle a little meat and milk, there is no reason for you to stop consuming it completely. However, controlling the amount of non-vegetarian food items you include can help you to keep a healthy heart and have a ton of other benefits, which is why it is recommended in the alkaline diet.

Apart from the obvious reasons in helping alkalize your body, veganism is also beneficial in various other ways. Here are a few reasons why doctors believe veganism is a healthy lifestyle.

### *Rich In Nutrients*

Although a lot of people believe that non-vegetarian food items are high in protein and can manage to provide your body with all the necessary nutrients required to keep the body healthy, veganism is actually healthy and is based on the nutrient levels of food.

When you consume a high non-vegetarian diet, the only thing you are providing your body with is protein. A vegan diet, on the other hand, comprises of whole foods that not only include high levels of fiber and antioxidants but also contain Vitamin A, C, E, B and Folic acids as well as potassium and magnesium.

If you want your vegan diet to work in your favor, you need to check the nutrient content of every meal you consume to make sure you give your body everything that it needs. While vegan diets are high in antioxidants and Vitamin E and C, you also need to have enough iron and calcium intake so that you get stronger bones. There are tons of vegan food that are high in iron and banana is a classic example.

### *It Helps In Weight Loss*

A number of people who suffer from obesity and weight issues are usually non-vegetarian. They have a higher content of fat in comparison to a vegan diet. If you follow a controlled diet and ensure you eat right, you will manage to lose weight faster compared to any other diet plan you choose to follow. When you combine veganism with an alkaline diet, not only does it boost your weight loss process, it also helps you to feel better and regularizes your blood sugar level thereby lowering the risk of diabetes.

### Low Risk Of Cancer

According to the World Health Organisation, controlling what you eat plays a huge role in lowering the risk of cancer. Acidic foods and non-vegetarian foods are right at the top of high-risk foods. They are more prone to causing cancer in comparison to fresh fruits and vegetables which are consumed by vegans on a regular basis.

### Lowers The Risk Of Heart Disease

Vegan are less prone to heart conditions and heart diseases in comparison to those who do not follow a vegan diet. The cholesterol level in a vegan is always lower than one who eats meat, and cholesterol is one of the leading reasons for heart-related problems. This is why a vegan diet is highly recommended if you have high cholesterol levels. Vegans also consume a lot of whole grains which work extremely well in promoting good heart health.

### *Reduces Arthritis Pain*

If you suffer from arthritis, then probiotic rich and raw vegan food can work wonders to lower the painful effect that it causes. Based on recent research, people who switched from a non-vegetarian diet to a natural whole food vegan diet for a span of 6 weeks managed to note a higher energy level and better functionality in comparison to other arthritis patients. The diet helps in greatly reducing joint swelling and stiffness, including pain that is common with rheumatoid arthritis and joint pain.

Before you plan a vegan diet, you need to understand that there are various kinds of foods in the diet plan which you should and shouldn't include. To figure out which food is healthy for you and which is not, you have to learn the alkaline content in the food. Vegan foods that have high acidic content should always be avoided because this is not going to benefit your body in any way. While vegan food is good, combining it with an alkaline diet is what plays a key role in helping you lose weight and fighting off diseases effectively.

# Chapter 3 - Benefits Of Alkalinity

An alkaline diet is all about increasing the alkalinity in your body to help you lead a healthy and long life that's disease free. This diet plan has been making waves in the market because of the effectiveness that it has to offer and more and more people are now planning to get used to the diet plan.

One of the major reasons why the alkaline diet has gained so much popularity is because it helps people get slim; however, that's not the only thing that alkalinity can help you with. Once you understand how alkalinity works and what it does to your body, you will never want to switch back to a diet plan that contains a high acid content.

## Protects Bone Density and Muscle Mass

Research has proven that high acid content in your body can affect your bones as well as your muscles. The reason it is important for you to focus on alkaline meals is because it increases the mineral intake in your body and focuses on better bone structure, resulting in lesser brittle bones. The acid content in your body is responsible for bone problems including joint pain and arthritis. When you lower the acid contents in your body, it gets easier for your bones to become stronger and absorb the healthy minerals that contribute towards better bone health. An alkaline diet focuses on increasing the production of vitamin D absorption in the bone and this is responsible for keeping your bones healthy. It also helps in the production of growth hormone and in ensuring that your body gets more strength from the minerals consumed. This helps effectively increase muscle mass and strength.

By increasing the alkalinity in your body, not only do you get better bones and better muscle strength but your endurance increases and you manage to exercise more effectively. This is vital for your overall health and it helps to keep away a number of bone-related diseases. When you have strong muscles, your body stays firmer and you age more gracefully.

## Lowers Risk for Hypertension and Stroke

Following an alkaline diet has a lot of anti-aging effects on the body. Apart from helping to protect muscle mass, it also decreases inflammation in the body and this works well to relieve a lot of stress and enhances cardiovascular health. People who follow an alkaline diet are less prone to hypertension and cholesterol. One of the leading causes of stroke is high cholesterol levels and blood clots caused by this cholesterol content. When you start an alkaline diet, your cholesterol level falls into place and it also helps to regulate blood pressure which is responsible for hypertension.

When you relieve stress, you start leading a healthy life not only physically but mentally as well. Stress is directly related to memory loss and a number of brain-related illnesses including Alzheimer's disease and Dementia. When you consume an alkaline based diet, you lower the risk of these diseases, and also prevent the risk of a heart attack and high blood pressure.

Alkaline-based diets also work really well on your vital organs including your kidneys. Kidney stones can be excruciatingly painful.

One of the major causes of kidney stone is the acid content in your body and when this content is reduced, you lower the risk.

## Lowers Chronic Pain and Inflammation

It's no secret that some women suffer from severe menstrual cramps during their menstruation while others manage to handle it more effectively. The leading cause of cramps during menstruation is high acid levels in the body. When you begin following an alkaline based diet, you reduce the risk of suffering from painful cramps because it helps soothe the muscles and relax them.

Alkalinity also helps prevent chronic back pain, muscle spasms, headache, inflammation, and joint pains. By simply reducing the acid levels in your body, you can keep a number of these problems at bay. When your body is healthier, you have more energy and you are able to get a lot more done during the day. It is important for you to have relaxed muscles and keep away inflammation and chronic pain to start leading a healthy lifestyle. This is where alkalinity comes into the picture and this is why it's so important.

## Boosts Vitamin Absorption and Prevents Magnesium Deficiency

Magnesium deficiency is highly underrated and people don't understand the importance of getting adequate magnesium in your body. When you fail to provide your body with the right amount, a lot of enzymes in your system begin dysfunctioning and it's not possible for your body to carry out its regular processes effectively. Lack of magnesium is one of the main causes of heart diseases and muscle spasms. It is also responsible for headache, sleep anxiety, and insomnia. When your magnesium levels are optimum, it also helps in activating Vitamin D and boosts the absorption of this vitamin into your bones for healthier and stronger bones. Magnesium also works well with other vitamins and helps the body get the benefits of those vitamins by absorbing it more effectively.

## Helps Improve Immune Functionality and Cancer Protection

One of the major benefits of alkalinity is that it helps oxidize your body more effectively and dispose of waste material faster. Apart from helping boost your metabolism level, it also strengthens the immune system to get rid of the dirty toxins on a regular basis. When you have a stronger immune system, your body manages to fight off bacteria and infections better. An alkaline diet contains high antioxidant properties responsible for fighting off the free radical cells mainly responsible for cancer cells growing in the system. An alkaline diet can help reduce the risk of cancer by killing these cells.

People who have multiple health problems should move to an alkaline based diet because not only does this help your body cope with medical treatments but it also helps you respond to the treatment better and encourages healing. Research has proven that chemotherapy works better when your pH levels are well balanced.

## Can Help You Maintain a Healthy Weight

One of the major reasons why an alkaline-based diet has gained so much popularity is because it helps burn fat and bring you back in shape. Unlike other diet plans that promise you effective results in just 30 days, this diet plan helps you to stay fit and active and helps you to fight off diseases which are most important. When you shift from an acid-based diet to an alkaline diet, you automatically start lowering the amount of calories you consume and this helps your body burn fat faster. It also helps your body to get stronger and it gives you more energy.

# Chapter 4 - Best Alkaline Foods

A common misconception about an alkaline based diet is that you need to simply shift to a vegan lifestyle and you start getting healthy. Although vegan food is good, in order for you to increase the alkalinity in your body, you have to consume foods that have high alkaline content.

**Fresh Fruits And Vegetables**

Following an effective alkaline diet entails including as much fruit and vegetable as possible. These fruits and vegetables work really well to balance the pH level in your body, making you healthier and more active. There is a variety you can purchase from the market but not all of these are great for alkaline diets. Here is a list of the most effective fruits and vegetables you should try to incorporate in your diet plan to increase alkaline levels in the body.

### *Avocado*

Avocado is an amazing fruit when you are on an alkaline diet. Not only does it help reduce acidic levels in your body, but it also provides you with a lot of nutrients such as vitamin B, E, C and K. It also has a high content of potassium and copper along with monounsaturated healthy fats. Avocado contains dietary fiber which is great for your metabolism and also works well to aid weight loss because it helps you feel fuller for longer.

### *Broccoli*

Although this vegetable isn't a favorite for a lot of people, including broccoli in your meals can give you a number of benefits. Broccoli is one of the few vegetables that are packed with nutrients that include Vitamin B6, K and C. It also has a high content of magnesium folate, Phosphorus Selenium and potassium that help diminish the acidic effects in your body and boost the alkaline content. It is always best to eat the vegetable raw.

### Celery

Celery has high Vitamin B and C content. It also offers anti-inflammatory and antioxidant properties which help to enhance cardiovascular functionality. Celery helps to fight oxidative stress, keeping your body relieved and enhancing muscle mass as well as relaxing your muscles and your brain. Celery is a great vegetable to prevent dehydration since it has a lot of water content. The vegetable also has a lot of folate and potassium.

## Cucumber

If there is one vegetable that can keep you hydrated all day long it's cucumber. Cucumber contains 96% water that helps increase your alkaline level and also releases your body of all the dirty toxins built up inside. Cucumbers are a rich source of vitamins and minerals such as Silicon, potassium and magnesium.

### Lemon

Although a lot of people believe that lemon has high acidic content, the truth is it is actually alkaline that's inside the lemon. This citrus fruit works wonders on your digestive system and also help in better nutrition absorption. When making a salad, squeeze a generous amount of lemon on your meal and you will manage to absorb the nutrients in the salad a lot better. Vitamin C also helps to boost your immunity and protect your body against a number of illnesses because of the high Vitamin C content in it.

### Peppers

Peppers are a great way to add flavor and color to your food. Whether you purchase green, yellow, or red bell peppers, they all have equal health benefits and provide you with a lot of Vitamin C and A. Peppers are also a great source of dietary fiber. Peppers contain a lot of antioxidants which help protect your body against cancer free radical cells.

### Spinach

If Popeye taught you anything, it's to eat as much spinach as you can. This leafy vegetable has a high nutrient profile and it provides your body with vitamins A, C, B2 and K. It also contains high levels of iron, magnesium, manganese, folate, as well as iron. Another great benefit of eating spinach is that it helps improve the alkaline-acid ratio in your body.

## All Raw Foods

The alkaline diet works best when you include raw food in your diet. The diet works well because you have kept the complete nutrition intact that the food has to offer. Whether it is in the shape of a salad, a soup or a smoothie, incorporate as much raw food as you can to boost your alkalinity and get healthier than ever before. One of the major reasons why you need to eat your food raw is because it's in the natural form and natural ingredients work best with alkalinity. When you cook your ingredients, it tends to lose a lot of the nutrients and it will not benefit your body as much as you would like it to. Some fruits and leafy vegetables have a high antioxidant content that are lost the minute it hits the heat. This is why you should try to incorporate as much raw food as possible in your diet. The best part about an alkaline diet is that you have a wide range of fruits and vegetables to choose from and these are best enjoyed raw.

**Alkaline Water**

When you adopt an alkaline diet, the one thing you need to learn is to prepare alkaline water. Alkaline water is nothing but water that has its alkaline levels boosted up to benefit you better. This water works wonders on your body and it helps to keep you healthy. One of the best things about alkaline water is that it has more hydrating properties in comparison to normal water, which means if you exercise or your body requires more water, the molecules in alkaline water can help rehydrate your body a lot faster than normal water.

Since the alkaline levels in the water are increased, it also boosts your immunity system and helps to fight off bacteria and infections more effectively. Regular consumption of alkaline water can work well to enhance your diet and take off all environmental toxins including stress. Unlike normal water, alkaline water contains a lot of magnesium and calcium and this contributes towards healthy bones. Since it has high antioxidant content, it also takes care of free radical cells and lowers the risk of cancer. Apart from fighting off diseases, alkaline water can also reverse the signs of aging and give you beautiful skin and hair. One of the best things about alkaline water is that it helps to lower the acidity in the system and it keeps your stomach and gastrointestinal tract healthy.

# Green Drinks / Smoothies

Greens have become an integral part of your diet and they should be included in every form possible. While we have seen the benefits of including raw greens in your daily diet, including green drinks or green smoothies can also benefit your physical health in a number of ways. Here are a few benefits of green smoothies that you probably didn't know about.

### Healthy Mentality

Green smoothies help you have a very positive and healthy frame of mind. The human mind is very difficult to train and it thrives on consistency. This means that if you start one particular habit that is healthy, your mind will start encouraging you to start another healthy habit. Try adding kale to your smoothie and see the mental change that it brings about. You will then want to take up a Yoga class that you have always wanted to try or go for a run on a daily basis when your smoothie intake is green.

### Reduce Unhealthy Cravings

When you start consuming a green smoothie on a daily basis, you will feel nourished and not crave for unhealthy sweets or foods. This can again be tied to the mental frame of mind where your mind will want to continue the healthy transformation and encourage you to eat healthy snacks. Green smoothies are a great way to cut down on the binge eating and reduce the number of unhealthy snacks that you consume daily.

### Glowing Skin

Since greens are rich in antioxidants, it does have a positive impact on your skin and you will see that your skin is hydrated and even the signs of aging have reduced.

### Healthy Heart

As you are already aware, greens are rich in antioxidants and they help to lower your cholesterol and keep away heart-related problems.

### Immunity Boost

Greens help boost your immune system and it will keep you away from illnesses for as long as you are consuming them. Consuming a green smoothie on a daily basis will keep you healthier than others who do not.

### Better Digestion

Since smoothies utilize whole veggies, there is a lot of fiber that you receive and this will help improve your digestion.

## Nutrient Absorption

When you consume smoothies daily, you will receive a lot of nutrients from vegetables such as spinach, kale, and lettuce.

### Better Energy

When you start absorbing a lot of nutrients every day, your energy levels will be very high and you will feel very invigorated.

## Other Foods

It's confusing to differentiate between foods that are highly acidic or alkaline, and that's the reason why people who just start out on an alkaline diet often end up eating the wrong kind of food. Just because something is vegan doesn't necessarily mean it is alkaline and it could benefit you. When you are on an alkaline diet, you should try and include alkaline fruits, nuts, legumes, and veggies. You should try to avoid foods that have high acid levels such as meat, poultry, fish, dairy, eggs, grains, and alcohol.

However, make sure that the fruits, nuts, legumes, and vegetables you include in your diet are highly alkaline and can promote the benefits of following the diet. There are some amazing alkaline foods that you should try to incorporate in your diet apart from the regular list that you will come across. These include soy products such as soya bean, miso, tofu, and tempeh. You can also look for unsweetened varieties of yogurt and curd as well as milk. Although some diets suggest that potatoes need to be avoided, you can most definitely include a small portion of potatoes when you are on an alkaline diet. You can also try to use as many herbs and spices to add flavor to your food.

# Chapter 5 - Alkaline Herbs And Supplements

If you thought going on an alkaline diet means you need to avoid adding flavor to your food, then you couldn't be more wrong. As long as it's healthy, you can use all kinds of spices and herbs to flavor your meal. The best part of an alkaline diet is you will find a wide range of herbs and supplements that you can use in your favor.

## Herbs

Following an alkaline diet could get difficult because of the number of food items you need to stop consuming especially when you are used to being a non-vegetarian. However, when you look at the bright side of things, there are tons of herbs you can add to your meals to add flavor and make it more palatable. Here are some herbs that not only add flavor but also work wonders with your health.

### Cayenne Pepper

Cayenne peppers add an amazing flavor to your food and while this is a pungent herb, it seems to be gaining a lot of popularity due to its taste. It has a lot of anti-inflammatory properties that work well to treat headaches and arthritis. It is also known to help reduce the signs of cancer. Cayenne pepper has also been associated with weight loss.

### Dandelion Greens

Dandelion Greens can add amazing flavor to your salad and you can also use it to make herbal tea. It has high alkaline properties and is known to treat kidney stones effectively.

## Turmeric

The bright yellow spice which is known to favor a number of curries has amazing properties and is also known to treat arthritis, cancer, and diabetes. It has a lot of medicinal properties and has been used by people for decades. If you can get your hands on fresh turmeric (the ones that look like ginger), you can use it not just to flavor your food but to make pickle and consume it with your meals. This works well to control your sugar levels and keep your bones healthy.

## Garlic

The amazing antifungal and antibiotic properties that garlic has can help heal your body from within very effectively. Garlic is an amazing antioxidant and it also helps fight parasites in the body and making you stronger.

Garlic is also known to be great for the heart and has high alkaline properties.

## Supplements

Although there are a number of foods that can help increase the levels of alkaline in your body, sometimes you need a little assistance and in this situation, supplements play a vital role. Here are a few supplements that you may be advised to take depending on the kind of diet plan you follow.

### *Potassium Citrate and Magnesium Citrate*

For alkalization to kick in, you need to have high levels of potassium and magnesium citrate. This is so that it lowers the amount of urine that is passed out of your body and also helps to enhance bone density and reduce the risk of brittle bones and fractures.

## Calcium

Calcium is an important supplement that you may want to start consuming when on an alkaline diet not only because it keeps your bones healthy, but it also helps in reducing hypertension.

## Glutamine

This supplement provides the body with amino acids which are necessary to lower the acidic levels and also helps to keep your kidney functioning effectively.

## Vitamin D

Without adequate vitamin D in your body, it will not manage to absorb calcium and magnesium effectively. This is why it's also important you consume this supplement through the food you are eating.

# Chapter 6 - Anti-Alkaline Foods And Habits

Starting off your alkaline diet might be tougher than you expected because of the various changes you need to make in your lifestyle in order to lower the acid levels and bring up your alkaline levels to an optimum level. There are various things that happen to your body when the acid levels are high and to bring this in control, it's necessary that you change your eating habits. The reason an alkaline diet is so necessary is because it helps reduce inflammation in the body which is one of the leading causes of various diseases including arthritis, diabetes, and cancer. It also causes chronic fatigue, irritability, unnecessary food cravings, and digestive problems. If you want to lead a healthy life and look great, it's important to address the root cause of all these problems which is high acid content in the body.

Once you bring your pH levels to the optimum level, it benefits you a great deal and you start feeling better about yourself. Not only do you manage to lose weight but you also feel more energetic and you drive away a number of illnesses. If you are diabetic, you will notice your sugar levels are in control and you will manage to get more done in a day because you simply feel great.

To follow a healthy alkaline diet, make sure you avoid meat and fish, food that contains any dairy product, eggs, alcohol, or nicotine and drugs, as well as refined grains of processed food. You should also try and stay away from any food items that have high sugar content as this isn't good for your body. Packaged cereal is also something you may want to avoid along with fast food. These foods have high acid levels and are not recommended during an alkaline diet.

Although alkaline diets do not recommend it, you avoid roasted nuts and seeds, tofu, tempeh, and soya bean in any form. It is highly recommended that you control eating these food items and never eat them more than twice a week. Food items that include vinegar or apple cider can be included in your diet more often since it's high alkaline. Avoid processed chocolates and dry fruits which have sugar added to it. Readymade salad dressings should also be limited since they are not great to consume on a daily basis.

If you want to train your mind to eat healthily, you need to take small steps and start with a few changes at a time so that your body gets used to it. If you are a hardcore non-vegetarian and you eat meats 5 to 6 times a week, do not give it up completely but instead decrease the size and limit your intake until you are comfortable giving it up and following an alkaline diet. An important rule to follow when choosing a diet plan, irrespective of which one it is, is to not force your body and make sure that whatever you plan on doing, your body is fine with it.

## High-Sodium Foods: Processed Foods

Processed foods are unhealthy, which is why they should be avoided completely whether or not you are on an alkaline diet. One of the major reasons why they are so bad is because most processed foods are loaded with sugar that adds unnecessary calories in your body and doesn't benefit you in any way. Processed foods contain no fiber content which means they affect your digestion and they don't work well for your metabolism levels as well.

Processed foods are highly addictive and this means that once you get hooked on to eating these foods, it is going to be difficult for you to stop. They are known to cause mood swings and they can lead to irritability and sometimes put you in a depressed state of mind. Most processed foods have high sodium content that is not healthy for you and is known to increase blood pressure. Processed food also interferes with your sleeping habits, making it difficult for you to get sound sleep. Since these food items are made to last long, they are loaded with preservatives which could take a longer time to digest and eventually lead to a lot of weight gain.

## Cold Cuts And Conventional Meats

When you lead a hectic life, cold cuts could work as a savior as they are just sitting in the freezer waiting for you to pull out and make a sandwich or a quick meal out of it. What most people don't realize is cold cuts are generally the main cause of health-related problems including high blood pressure, obesity, and high cholesterol. Cold cuts are cured meats which are preserved either by salting or smoking, and in some cases are preserved with chemicals such as sodium nitrate, all of which have high health risks. They have a lot of unnecessary calories and should be avoided if you want to lead a healthy life. Reducing the amount of cold cuts in your diet can help reduce the risk of cancer, according to the World Health Organisation.

## Processed Cereals

Processed cereals are easy to use for people who are always on the rush. The problem with processed cereal is that it either has a lot of sugar content or the ones that are low on sugar levels contain artificial sweeteners, both of which are highly acidic for the body. These contain toxic ingredients that only destroy your body over time and don't benefit you in any way. They do not have any nutrients and only keep you full for a couple of hours before your body starts craving for more junk food.

## Eggs

Eggs are a controversial subject when it comes to following an alkaline diet because an alkaline diet asks you to avoid it completely. While they usually say that an egg is healthy, the truth is consuming it may not be as beneficial as you imagine them to be. While they are high in protein content, eggs also contain a lot of cholesterol which is not great for your system and can increase the risk of a heart attack and clogged arteries. High cholesterol levels are often linked with liver cancer which is why you may want to avoid eating an egg if you want to keep your liver healthy. It is also believed that eggs contain chlorine, a compound that is highly toxic and starts growing in the gut of the person thereby increasing the risk of various health conditions. Eggs are also known to be highly acidic which affects the alkaline levels in your body and causes multiple health issues.

## Caffeinated Drinks and Alcohol

Drinks that have high caffeine form bubbles in the stomach causing it to expand and giving you the feeling of bloatedness. This is an uncomfortable feeling not only because you start feeling sick, but also because it affects your digestive system. Foods that contain caffeine and aerated drinks are highly acidic and should be avoided when you are on an alkaline diet and trying to get healthy. These drinks are also often loaded with a lot of sugar which adds unnecessary calories to your diet.

When you start an alkaline diet, the first thing you need to get out of your list is alcohol because alcohol is highly acidic and it could increase the amount of gastric acid in your system. The worst part about alcohol is people start consuming it with a number of carbonated drinks that multiplies the problem and creates uncomfortable situations for your body. Alcohol is not good for your liver and people who drink are more prone to liver-related issues including enlargement of the liver and cirrhosis of the liver, both of which can be avoided by cutting down on your alcohol consumption. Let's not forget, alcohol and caffeine interfere with your pH balance and push you more towards the acidic side.

## Oats and Whole Wheat Products

Oats and whole wheat may sound amazing to consume when you are on a diet but these are also food products you may want to avoid when you switch to an alkaline diet. Although oats and whole wheat are healthy, the problem with both these items is that they are complex carbohydrates that take a longer time to break down in your body, thereby making it difficult for the body to digest the food. This increases the acid levels in your system and makes it difficult to maintain a healthy pH balance when you are trying to get your body's alkaline levels high.

## Milk

As a child, you were told you should drink a glass of milk to make your bones healthy. The truth however, is that cow's milk actually takes off the Calcium from your bones. While calcium is an amazing acid neutralizer, milk isn't and it tends to add more acid to your body than you can imagine. This means every time you drink a glass of milk, your body is drained of the calcium content thereby increasing the acid levels. Several researchers have proven that milk can lead to prostate cancer which is why people should switch to soy milk instead. Your body needs a lot of time to digest milk and if it isn't digested properly, it could lead to bloating, diarrhea, and cramps that could make you uncomfortable.

Milk also has a lot of cholesterol, and regular consumption can increase your cholesterol levels quite a bit. Research has proven that people who consume more milk are more prone to ovarian cancer. If you have heard that you should only use antibiotics when prescribed by a doctor and always complete the dosage so that your body does not start building a resistance towards the medication, you may want to stay off milk because cow's milk contains antibiotics and they start entering your system the minute you drink it and creates an anti drug-resistant atmosphere in your body. You won't even know what drugs you are resistant to because you haven't consumed them directly. Milk is often linked to weight gain and people who drink milk on a regular basis tend to add more weight in comparison to those who don't. You can substitute milk with soy-based milk products that are healthy and more alkaline in nature.

**Peanuts and Walnuts**

While an alkaline diet asks you to consume nuts on a regular basis, you need to stay away from peanuts and walnuts for a reason. Both peanuts and walnuts are known to increase the acid levels in your body and this is why you may want to stay away from them. These nuts interfere with the pH balance in your body and make it difficult for you to come to the level of alkalinity that you wish. These nuts are also known to create multiple health issues including congestion and interference in the detoxification process during an alkaline diet. Unlike most of the other nuts that help you to lose weight, peanuts and walnuts are generally associated with weight gain which is why you may want to stay away from them during your alkaline diet.

## Pasta, Rice, Bread and Packaged Grain Products

If you are starting an alkaline diet, the one thing you have to lay off is your pasta, rice, and bread for a reason. They are known to cause the number of dietary issues because of the heavy carbohydrates and starch content that they have. These increase the acidity in your body and are known to cause gas and heat burn along with bloating. They are also known to release complex sugars which are difficult to digest and gets accumulated as fat in your body.

## The Kind Of Habits That Can Cause Acidity In Your Body

If you are going on an alkaline diet, it isn't just about what you eat but also what you need to avoid to get healthy. If you want your alkaline diet to go well, you need to identify the biggest offender of the diet and stay as far away from them as possible.

### *Alcohol and Drugs*

We have already understood that alcohol has high acid content which is why you should avoid it. Alcohol has many underlying effects as well such as causing depression and stress on a person. The problem with alcohol is that it's addictive and just like drugs, it could make you lethargic and lazy. Drugs are also high in acid content and when you start consuming drugs or start smoking on a regular basis, you are increasing the acid content in your body. If you want to follow a healthy alkaline diet, you need to cut off the alcohol and stop smoking or stop consuming drugs in any form.

### High Caffeine Intake

Caffeine in any form should be avoided because it interferes with the functionality of your body and increases your heart rate unnecessarily. Caffeine also has high acid content along with a lot of unwanted sugar which results in weight gain. Consuming too many caffeine products will interfere with your sleeping habit and this causes stress as well as improper functionality of the organs.

### Antibiotic Overuse

When you start popping pills unnecessarily, this does not benefit you in any way and it makes your body so used to those medicines that they won't work even when you actually have an infection that needs to be treated. These infections are known as drug-resistant infections and they are only caused when you abuse antibiotics and consume them over your recommended amount. Too much antibiotics also result in acid reflux and high acidity levels in your body which has a number of side effects and affects your alkaline diet.

### Artificial Sweeteners

Artificial sweeteners are highly acidic and interfere with the process of an alkaline diet. If you want to stay healthy, you have to learn to avoid your cravings for sweets and this includes artificial sweeteners. The best artificial sweeteners are registered as low as 2.5 on a pH balance scale meaning that they are extremely acidic. If you continue using artificial sweeteners in your diet, you will not manage to bring your pH balance to the alkaline level you desire and the diet will not work as planned.

### Chronic Stress

High stress level usually results in acidity and acid reflux, which is why it's important for you to learn how to relax and calm your body before you take on an alkaline diet. If you suffer from serious stress, it is going to be very difficult for you to control your acid levels in the body and this could mean that following the diet may not benefit you in the way you want, no matter how many alkalizing foods you consume. If you are going through too much stress, the best thing to do would be to consult a doctor and bring your stress levels in control before you start the diet plan.

To get the best out of your alkaline diet, it's important that you learn how to identify acidic food items and stay away from them. Apart from that, here are some basic tips you may want to follow in order to make the most out of the alkaline diet plan and lead a healthy life.

## Eat Regularly

It is important for you to make time to eat regular and healthy meals if you want your body to get into control. No matter how busy you are, try to make time to ensure you eat the right amount of food multiple times a day rather than stuffing too much food two or three times a day.

## Sleep Well

If you want to get healthy and want the alkaline diet to work, you need to provide your body with enough rest every day. You should try and get at least seven to eight hours of sleep because this helps relax your body and also relieves your body from a lot of acids, making you feel unhealthy.

## Stop Smoking

If you want the alkaline diet to work, you need to say goodbye to your smoking habit so that it benefits you and you manage to make the diet a successful one. This will not only help you in weight loss but will also drive away diseases and increase your energy levels.

## Low Levels of Nutrients in Foods Due to Industrial Farming

When you start to follow an alkaline diet, the one thing you may want to focus on is purchasing products that are organic and homegrown. Products that are available on an industrial level do not contain the number of nutrients as you would want them to because they are mass produced and usually chemical based. Thankfully, there are farmers markets that are available in every locality and if there is one close to you, make the most of it and purchase all fresh fruits and vegetables from a farmers market so that you get homegrown and organic food products.

## Low Levels of Fiber in the Diet

When you follow an alkaline diet, the one thing you need to make sure is that you provide your body with enough fiber so that it functions effectively and you manage to eliminate the dirty toxins that you are suffering from. If you want to lose weight during the alkaline diet, fiber plays an essential role in easing better digestion. Broccoli, apples, and carrots are high in fiber so when you start your diet, make sure to include plenty of these on a daily basis.

## Including Non Grass-Fed Animal Meats in the Diet

It is not easy for a non-vegetarian to switch to an alkaline diet that is completely vegan, and this is why you may want to cut down the amount of meat you include in your daily life without completely eliminating it. However, there are meats that are non grass-fed that you may want to try and avoid because these are higher in fat and calories. Grass-fed meat manages to provide you with proteins which benefit you. While your goal should be to give up on meat completely, you can always start by reducing the amount of meat you eat and choosing a flexitarian diet for a few days.

## Eliminating Unnecessary Hormones from Your Life

In order for you to stay healthy, it is important to identify your exposure to hidden hormones. These hormones could be found in a variety of food items and beauty products as well as plastics that you are often exposed to. The best way to understand where the hidden hormones lie is to check for the level of chemicals in the product because that's what usually relates to as a hidden hormone. If you want to lower the risk of exposure to these hidden hormones, you might want to try opting in for natural products, whether it's for food or your beauty products or even plastic and try to limit the amount of chemicals in your life.

## Radiation

Electromagnetic radiation can cause a number of side effects in your life and while we believe we keep ourselves away from this exposure, the truth is there are a number of products you use on a daily basis including your cell phone and your microwave that release this radiation more than you would like them to. If you want to stay healthy, you should try to stop heating food in a microwave and make smaller portions that you finish up in one consumption. You should also sleep away from your cell phone so that it does not affect you while you sleep.

## Preservatives in Food Coloring

While natural food coloring is still manageable, artificial food colors are full of chemicals and preservatives which do not work well on your body and may slow down the process of digestion. This also affects your vital organs which is why you should stay away from any product that has preservatives or artificial food coloring.

## Pesticides

Pesticides are harmful to the environment and while a lot of people know this, what they don't realize is these pesticides can also be extremely harmful to the human body as well. Prolonged exposure to pesticides can lead to various health-related issues and can increase the risk of cancer. If you believe organic is something that is just a little more expensive, then you may want to reconsider because too much of pesticides could increase neurological disorders such as Parkinson's disease, leukemia, asthma, and other diseases in your body. An alkaline diet always recommends raw, organic and natural foods as a force to the ones that are treated with pesticides for the obvious reasons.

## Over-Exercise

It's common for people to feel pumped once they start any diet plan and they always like to accompany it with an exercise regime. While exercise is great, it's important for you to make sure you don't overdo it because an excess of anything will be bad and that is also true for exercise. If you attempt exercising more than your body can handle, you could end up with a muscle tear or tissue damage that could take months to heal. Instead of doing too much on one day, you may want to start slow but make sure that you don't miss a single day of exercise so that your body gets movement regularly and you manage to burn fat and increase your energy levels effectively.

## Pollution

Although it is hard to stay away from pollution, this is something that could affect your body in various ways on a regular basis. High pollution levels can cause damage to your lungs, brain, and heart. The reason why an alkaline diet is recommended is because this helps clean your organs and increases the strength of your lungs as well as cleanses your heart and removes all the dirty toxins and pollutants from your body regularly.

## Poor Chewing and Eating Habits

One of the worst things that you can do is to eat your food too quickly. The faster you swallow, the higher the chances of you staying overweight because it takes a while for bigger food particles to digest in the body as compared to smaller particles that you chew properly. It is also said that you should eat your food slower because this gives your body enough time to digest the food more effectively and drinking water in between your meals definitely helps you to stay fitter in comparison to those who start chewing and swallowing the food really fast.

## Shallow Breathing

Most people lead a hectic life and they literally have no time to take a deep breath! If you want to stay healthy, it's important to breathe easily and with comfort rather than taking short breaths and trying to take in as much air in a short shallow breath as possible. The deeper your breaths are, the more relaxed your body is and the better it is for your lungs. In case you have a breathing problem and you are used to taking shorter breaths, you may want to start practicing taking deep breaths at least five to six times a day until you get into the habit of it.

# Chapter 7: Dr Sebi's 10 Day Cleanse

Dr. Sebi had introduced a 10 day cleanse that helps you eat healthy while keeping up with the demands of a busy lifestyle. There are a number of foods that are available on the go, however these foods will make your body very unhealthy and you will be filled with a lot of negative sensations. These foods such as red meat, fast food, and greasy foods lead to a lot of weight gain as well as health complications and heart problems.

Over a period of time, you will realize that your energy is considerably low and this is something that can be avoided with the help of Dr. Sebi's 10 day cleanse. If you are already too far ahead in terms of eating unhealthy foods and are not feeling great about your weight that you have put on, you may want to try this 10 day cleanse and it will help bring your body back on track. This 10 day cleanse helps to remove all the low energy from your body and it will also relieve you of the stress that you are going through.

## Understanding The 10 Day Cleanse

Following the 10 day cleanse is not as easy as it sounds and you need a lot of discipline in order to make sure that you get your body's balance back in place. The key to the 10 day cleanse is to make sure that you keep away from all kinds of acidic foods and you drink natural spring water. There are four different ways that you can go about doing the Dr. Sebi 10 day cleanse. Here is what each of them comprises of.

### *Fasting*

One of the hardest ways to go about Dr. Sebi's 10 day cleanse is with fasting. While fasting may seem difficult, it is definitely the most effective when it comes to reversing various health conditions that you are undergoing. Before you try the option of fasting, you need to make sure that you consult your doctor and see if you are fit enough to go through with this process. The fasting process mainly focuses on eating sea moss and drinking spring water. Your food intake is severely limited during this cleansing process and it may be difficult to sustain it if your body is not strong enough.

### *Juice Cleanse*

As the name states, this is a juice cleansing process and you are able to consume all kinds of fruits and vegetables in their liquid form. If you feel that only juices may not keep you going, then you may want to add a bit of sea moss powder or sea moss gel after drinking your juice. This will ensure that you do not give in to your hunger temptations and you stay on track with the cleansing process. Before you go ahead with this cleansing process, you need to make sure that you invest in a blender that is very reliable as well as stable.

## *Food and Juice Cleanse*

This is definitely one of the best cleansers to make sure that you stay on track with the cleansing process and you achieve your weight loss goals. This cleanse recommends that you eat raw foods as much as possible; however if you are not able to do that, you should stick to the recommended foods by Dr. Sebi. The first few days of this cleanse are very difficult however, if you make it past the first four days, you will be able to complete the 10 days successfully. The best part about this cleanse is that you will not crave for any kind of junk food after just one week.

*Food, Juice as well as Herb Cleanse*

Adding herbs to your cleansing process can definitely help make the cleanse more effective. The reason a lot of people add herbs to their cleanse is it helps to remove all the toxins from the body and it will also improve the mindset of the person. The people that are on this cleanse can consume vegetable broth as well as all kinds of fruits and vegetable juices. You can even eat vegetables, fruits, nuts, salads, as well as grains. You need to make sure that everything you consume is fresh and natural as this will help to reset the balance of your body and remove all the toxins successfully.

## Enhancing The 10 Day Cleanse

While the 10 day cleanse is not very easy, you can enhance the cleanse further by adding herbs to it. Irrespective of the kind of cleanse you are doing, you can add herbs to your diet and this will take your cleanse to the next level. You can purchase herbal supplements that are available in capsule form and this will help you go through the day without having the need to rely on solid foods. A number of people that are on liquid cleanses often give up after the second day because they are not able to stay away from solid foods. These herbal supplements will help your body feel good and it will also help Dr. Sebi's cleansing process to be successful.

# Conclusion

With so many diet plans being introduced into the market on a regular basis, it is natural to get confused with regards to which one will work and which ones make absolutely no sense! If you are looking to lose weight without staying concerned about your health, then you should probably look for something that works fast and has no logic to it. While these kinds of diet plans often attract more customers, they are the kind of diet plans that eventually fail because they don't live up to their expectations and once somebody gives up the diet, they get back to the way they were or even heavier.

The reason an alkaline diet is so perfectly crafted is because it doesn't just focus on losing weight, but it also includes crucial steps that help reduce and reverse the risks of life-threatening diseases including cancer and diabetes. An alkaline diet is the only diet that can help cure you from within and you will feel better and more energetic in no time.

An alkaline diet may be difficult to start off with but once you start it, you will realize how amazing you feel and you'll never want to get off this diet plan in your life. One small step towards a healthy future can pave the path for a happy, stress-free, younger, energetic and beautiful you! Take that step today and adapt to an alkaline way of life!

Lightning Source UK Ltd.
Milton Keynes UK
UKHW020442080921
390192UK00013B/2815